KETO DIET FOR WOMEN OVER
UK Edition

Ultimate Cookbook with Tasty & Easy Recipes for a Healthy Life

4-Week Meal Plan to Jumpstart Your Weight Loss Journey

Table of Contents

Introduction 7

Chapter 1: Keto and You 10

    A Brief History of Keto 11

    Why Do You Choose a Keto Diet? 14

    Ketosis 16

Chapter 2: 11 Reasons Why Women Over 50 Should Try Keto 19

    1. Accelerates Metabolism 19

    2. Hormones Production 19

    3. Weight Loss 19

    4. Oxidative Stress 19

    5. Diabetes 20

    6. PCOS 20

    7. Cures Cancer 20

    8. Inflammation 20

    9. Athletic Performance with More Energy 21

    10. Decreased Cardiovascular Risk 22

    11. A Cure for Aging 22

Chapter 3: 7 Keto Diet Weight Loss Secrets 24

    1. Too Many Snacks 24

    2. Not Consuming Enough Fat 24

    3. Consuming Excessive Calories 24

    4. Consuming a lot of Protein 24

    5. Not Getting Enough Water 25

    6. Low on Electrolytes 25

    7. Consuming Hidden Carbs 26

Recipes for Breakfast 27
- Mayonnaise Waffles 28
- Coconut Macadamia Bars 30
- Turmeric Muffins 31
- Bacon Avocado Bombs 33
- Tofu & Mushroom Muffins 34
- Chicken, Bacon, Avocado Caesar Salad 36
- Shrimp and Olives Pan 37
- Baked Eggs 38
- Crêpes with Lemon-Buttery Syrup 39
- Yogurt Waffles 41
- Bacon Omelet 43
- Bell Pepper Frittata 45

Recipes for Lunch 47
- Broccoli and Turkey Dish 48
- Zucchini Sushi 49
- Easy Mayo Salmon 50
- Caprese Zoodles 51
- Zesty Avocado and Lettuce Salad 52
- Keto Buffalo Chicken Empanadas 53
- Pepperoni and Cheddar Stromboli 54
- Veggie, Bacon, and Egg Dish 55
- Hot Spicy Chicken 56
- Keto Teriyaki Chicken 57
- California Burger Bowls 58
- Parmesan Brussels Sprouts Salad 60

Dinner Recipes 61
- Broccoli and Chicken Casserole 62
- Crispy Peanut Tofu and Cauliflower Rice Stir-Fry 63
- Chicken Schnitzel 64
- Mexican Shredded Beef 65
- Creamy Chicken Bake 67
- Beef Stew 68
- Baked Jerked Chicken 70
- Simple Keto Fried Chicken 71
- Salmon & Shrimp Stew 72
- Sausage Stuffed Zucchini Boats 73
- Balsamic Steaks 75

Dessert Recipes 77
- Keto Sorbet 78
- Pumpkin Pie Cupcakes 79
- Brownies 80
- Ice Cream 81
- Fresh Berries with Cream 82
- Keto Brownies 83
- Keto Creamy Granola 84
- Keto Popsicle 85
- Special Keto Pudding 86
- Keto Cheesecakes 87
- Cocoa Brownies 88
- Raspberry and Coconut 90
- Keto Sorbet 91

    Chocolate Chip Cookies 92

4-Week Meal Plan 94

    Week 1 95

    Week 2 96

    Week 3 97

    Week 4 98

    BONUS: Approved Food List for The Ketotarian 99

Introduction

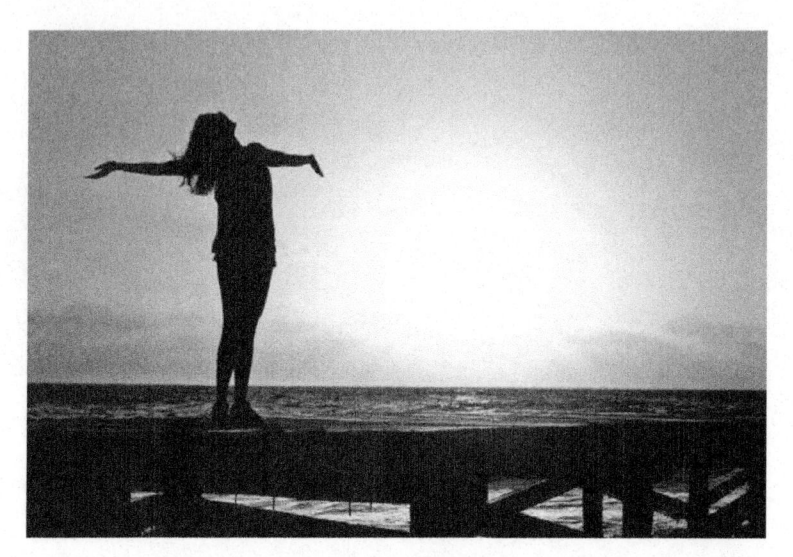

The woman's body, at any age, is an amazing thing. We begin as tiny babies and grow up to have babies ourselves. We can hold down a job, carry a pregnancy, nurture tiny humans, and take care of our mates—all at the same time! Any woman who has reached the glorious age of fifty, or even beyond, should celebrate. You have experienced more changes, especially in your body, than men ever will. Unfortunately, all of the things that make the woman a glorious creature can also work against her when trying to be healthy and active long into her senior years.

The first major experience a woman of fifty and over will experience is menopause. That monthly inconvenience will be gone forever, and you will be able to experience life without it.

But the joy of freedom from that monthly event can also mean an increase in developing belly fat and possibly other health consequences. That's because the onset of menopause means the cessation of your body's production of estrogen.

The estrogens in your body are the hormones that your body produces related to your sexual orientation. They are what make you a woman. The estrogens start and maintain the things that make you a woman—the breasts, the reproduction, and your monthly cycle.

All of the forms of estrogen have a particular responsibility in your body. One of the types that decrease dramatically in production after menopause is the one that helps you regulate your metabolism and keep your body weight under control.

This is why many women tend to accumulate fat around their midsections. This fat collects around their internal organs and is not only unattractive, but it is also dangerous. This visceral fat can lead to stroke, heart disease, diabetes, and some forms of cancer. And older women often tend to move less than they did when they were younger.

Since they no longer have children to chase, and many no longer work, they find themselves with less reason to move and more excuses to sit. Unfortunately, this not only leads to weight gain but also the stiffening of their joints.

Young women often have poor dietary habits but do not gain weight because the estrogens help them to keep their metabolism running high. This also helps to keep the level of cholesterol in the blood at a normal level. When you pass fifty, cholesterol levels begin to rise, and if they rise too high, you might be at an increased risk of heart attacks and strokes. Cholesterol is made naturally by the body. The body will make the amount that it needs for its normal functions. When processed foods, sugary foods, and unhealthy fats are consumed regularly, they will cause a buildup of excess cholesterol, which will lead to the formation of plaque in your arteries.

Part of the problem with the older woman's joints is the excess weight that she is carrying around. Being overweight puts enormous strain on the lower body joints, causing them to wear faster than they normally would.

Weight gain comes from consuming a diet that is high in processed foods and excess sugar, which will lead to obesity, which will lead to joint pain and deterioration. On the more serious side, all of this indulgence can lead to the development of osteoporosis, which can begin with the loss of estrogen and be made worse by excess weight and lack of exercise.

A degenerative condition where your bones become more porous and stop regenerating happens when you get older and known as osteoporosis. It is the main reason why older people, especially women who tend to have smaller bones than men, often suffer hip fractures from falls. In osteoporosis, the bone can't grow quickly enough to replace what is deteriorating.

It is normal for your muscles to lose some of their natural elasticity and strength as you age, simply because the muscles are getting older, and you are not moving as much. But maintaining good muscle tone is the key to keeping you moving throughout the remainder of your life and living it since the loss of muscle strength is the biggest reason many older adults find themselves unable to take care of themselves.

Strong muscles will help to keep you from falling. You need them to help reduce pain in your joints, keep your weight at a healthy level, and help to keep your bones strong and functional.

While it is not possible to stop the effects of aging, you can minimize them and keep yourself healthy and active far into the future by mixing a combination of exercise with the right kind of diet to give you the nutrients you need. And that diet is the keto diet.

I also experienced those parts of my life feeling unhealthy. I tried almost everything, even drugs, and nothing worked for me, except for the last four weeks, I discovered a natural method that is quick, simple, and straightforward that immediately developed my body with 100 percent natural. Since I discovered the keto diet, it is very rewarding and fun to eat and enjoy such wonderful healthy food. I started a keto diet on December 26 last year and lost 15 kilos by this time. It is great, and I feel great. I want to lose 25 kilos more to remain healthy and live a lot of time with my husband. I love to travel with him, and we travel to many places around the world. Suppose you are interested in losing weight, healthy eating, and living a healthy and long life. In that case, I recommend you to try the keto diet to overcome your obesity problem.

Chapter 1: Keto and You

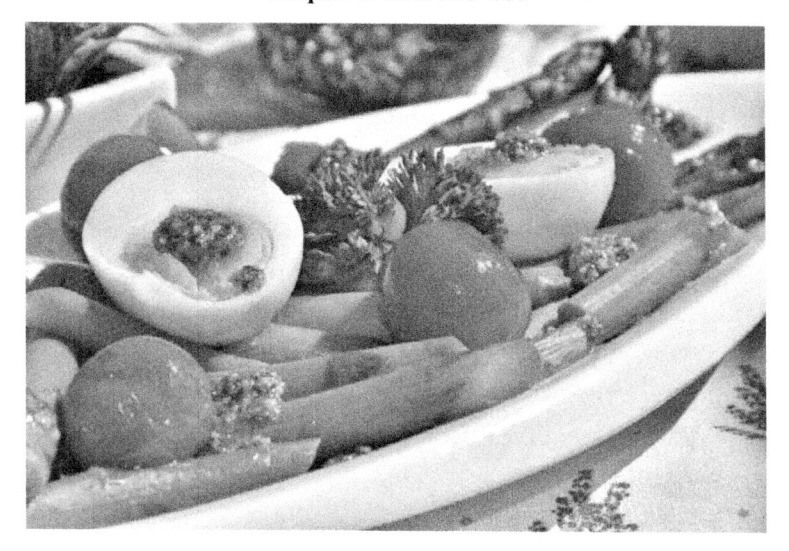

You have starvation, extreme diets, and exercise. You may have enjoyed some success but found that you could not attain your ultimate goals. Maybe you ended up backtracking with your weight loss because the diets were not sustainable or realistic. Perhaps you were just plain miserable. Keto returns you to the metabolic state your ancestors enjoyed, the way you were meant to live with. Keto happens quickly in humans. It allows you to wake up refreshed even if you have not eaten for the past twelve hours. You are made for it.

The real world, where you lounge in chairs for half the day, has gotten in your way. You snack on something every two to three hours. You eat carbs that you do not need for the energetic pursuits you do not pursue. You eat from morning to night. After your five or six hours of sleep, you grab junk food and a flavored coffee on the way to school or work. You are overfed. You exist in a permanently fed state. Ketosis is not a state that many people have experienced since people seem never to stop eating.

A Brief History of Keto

As far back as the ancient physicians in Greece, we have been told that healthy weight can easily be maintained by restricting calories from food. For centuries people fasted to treat various illnesses, particularly epilepsy. In the early twentieth century, doctors began experimenting with fasting to control the effects of epilepsy, in the days before medications were introduced. It was found that people who subscribed to the 'water diet' had fewer seizures and were sometimes considered 'cured.' As you can probably guess, the water diet consisted of water. And while people did enjoy a respite from seizures, it isn't easy to maintain a healthy lifestyle while consuming a diet made up of only water.

But this was an exciting time for medical discoveries as patients and physicians alike were beginning to wonder exactly what made the body function the way it did. An endocrinologist discovered that people who lived on the water diet secreted three compounds from their livers that were water-soluble, meaning they were flushed away by water. These three compounds together were called 'ketones.'

Since it was impossible to live on water for the remainder of a person's life, doctors began experimenting with different combinations of food so that their epileptic patients could eat. They discovered that a lower diet in carbohydrates and rich in fats with the right amount of protein would produce the same epilepsy-free results that the water diet did. Patients could consume a diet of specific foods that mimicked the effect of fasting on their bodies. Eating more fat and removing sugar from the diet caused the liver to release the body's ketones for energy. Physicians had already concluded that the ketones the body was releasing were the leading cause of epileptic seizures. Since the liver also released these on a high-fat, low-carb diet, they named this diet the ketogenic diet.

So, physicians used this diet with great success on children and adults who had epilepsy. Seizures lessened or stopped altogether, and people were able to resume everyday life. But then doctors began noticing that people, who followed the keto diet, the children especially, were displaying other changes in their bodies that went beyond the cessation of seizures. These people lost weight and were more active. Being more alert during the day helped them sleep better at night. The children were mostly more comfortable to discipline and much less irritable than before.

But eventually, anticonvulsant drugs were invented that allowed people with epilepsy to take medication and be free from the dietary plan restrictions. This reversal of thought was when refrigeration was still not widely used, so that following the constraints of the keto diet may have been difficult for many people. And taking a pill was so much easier. So, the keto diet was no longer taught in medical school and generally fell out of favor with most doctors until a prominent event in the latter part of the twentieth century that changed the way people looked at keto and brought it into the modern world.

At that time, a television producer and his wife looked for something to help their young son, who suffered from severe seizures. Even strong medications would not control the child's seizures that would often come one after the other. While doing internet research, his parents stumbled over a ketogenic diet description, which would eventually revolutionize their lives. When they started their young son on the keto diet, his seizures virtually vanished, and he was finally able to enjoy life as a normal little boy. A television movie soon followed, and the world was once again in love with the keto diet.

But even with its success in treating epilepsy, the keto diet would not have been thought of so favorably if it did not help people achieve and maintain an average healthy weight. And while the keto diet itself is relatively new, this eating style has been around since early man. Hunting and gathering was a way of life for our ancient ancestors. They hunted meat and gathered plants and berries as they traveled from place to place, hunting meat. And no part of the meat was wasted, which meant that early man also ate the fat piece of the meat and the lean part. As each generation has moved less and relied on processed foods, they have gradually become more obese and less healthy.

Enter the keto diet. Following the keto diet relies on a massive intake of fats, a moderate protein intake, and a low intake of carbohydrates to achieve weight loss and later maintain a healthy weight. The keto diet's primary function is to put your body into a ketosis state, causing your body to produce ketones that your body will use for energy instead of using the sugar from the foods you consume. A high carbohydrate diet will repress the body's ability to produce ketones, and the excess sugar gets stored as fat.

Why Do You Choose a Keto Diet?

When you eat the food you consume, it goes into your stomach, where acids and enzymes mix with the chewed food and break it down into even smaller particles. When your meal leaves your stomach, it has been liquefied for easier passage into and through the small intestine. In the small intestine, the body completes the job of digesting your food and begins to move it into your bloodstream to other parts of the body. While your gall bladder produces bile to help digest your food and your liver stores nutrients and filters out toxins, your pancreas is perhaps the next most crucial organ in the food use process. The pancreas is the main organ in your body that helps regulate your blood sugar levels through insulin production.

The pancreas' hormone insulin is made to help your body use glucose (sugar) from the food that you eat for energy. While the body needs this sugar for power, the sugar molecules do not pass into the cells themselves. They need to attach to molecules of insulin to be able to enter the cells. Your blood sugar rises when you eat. Your pancreas is alerted to release insulin to help carry the sugar into the cells to use the sugar for energy. The problem arises when people either overeat food or eat too many simple carbs that will turn into sugar in the body. When this happens, the body receives too many signals too often for increasing the level of insulin. Eventually, the cells will stop reacting to insulin because they are full of glucose and have no room for more. The excess glucose is stored in the body as excess body fat. When this happens, you now have two overwhelming problems, insulin resistance and obesity.

Many older women have a problem with excess belly fat, and the reason for this is simple. Your body stores extra glucose as fat, and the body will search for the most comfortable place to dump this glucose. The cavities of the midsection, around the abdomen's internal organs, are the perfect place – in the body's opinion – to dump off all of that excess sugar so it can turn into fat. The insulin turns the glucose into glycogen and stores it in your belly for possible future needs.

So it is a known fact that eating more food than you need for survival leads to obesity. By continuously overeating, you train your body to think that it needs food all day long, which is not valid. Many cultures worldwide discourage snacking between meals, and those people tend to live long, healthy lives. So you keep overeating, and then one day you realize that you have a body filled with little pockets of fat. You will need to rid your body of this excess fat by exercising regularly and consuming a healthy diet. And this is where the keto diet will be the most beneficial.

While keto is referred to as the 'keto diet,' it should not be considered a diet. No one should ever plan to live on a diet forever, as that implies restricting things, and we do not like to deprive ourselves. Instead, keto should be thought of as a way of life that you will follow to be healthy and fit. When you live the keto way of life, your body will start by breaking down excess fat and using these energy reserves. This cleansing is what the body does naturally during starvation; it uses stored fat to fuel the body when new food sources are not readily available.

Ketosis

Ketosis comes on anywhere from two days to one week after beginning the keto diet. This level is the goal of the keto diet to push your body into ketosis. Once you have reached a ketosis state, you will need to maintain the diet to remain in ketosis. Getting into ketosis is the worst side effect of the keto diet, but you will not regret your decision once you get past the initial stage. Ketosis is often referred to as keto flu because it feels much like you have viral flu. The symptoms of beginning ketosis are varied:

- Diarrhea
- Sleep disturbances
- Weakness during exercise and after
- Temporary loss of libido
- Exhaustion
- Cravings for sugary foods
- Headaches
- Bloating
- Irritability and moodiness
- Constipation
- Bad breath

The bad breath of ketosis is caused by waste products being eliminated from your body. These waste products are stored in fat cells and need to be eliminated as the fat cells are destroyed. Your body will eliminate waste through your breath, your sweat, or through defecation or urination.

You might naturally feel deprived of sugary treats when you begin the keto diet. We all love a good glazed doughnut or a massive bowl of cake and ice cream, and we miss these when they are gone. Just remember they are not gone forever, and there is plenty of satisfying dessert options on the keto diet. You will crave carbs because they taste good, but you will be consuming enough foods not to need the carbs to make up for the caloric intake. And decreasing carb intake may lead to a decrease in your ability to sleep well at night. Consuming carbs causes the brain to release hormones melatonin and serotonin, which are the hormones that make you sleepy and happy, respectively. Eventually, the keto diet will teach your body to release hormones at the proper times but in the meantime, try to keep a consistent sleep schedule even on your days off.

Some people will experience bloating, constipation, or diarrhea when beginning the keto diet. Food affects all people differently. Diarrhea comes from the increase in fats in your diet. The bloating is from the body, releasing toxins from the stored fats that are being digested. Constipation may also go along with increased urination. Fat cells are the primary sources of water storage in your body. When you begin eliminating fat cells, the excess water leaves your body in the form of perspiration or urination, leaving very little for the bowels to use for defecation. And less water in your body may lead to feelings of fatigue or muscle weakness.

Moodiness and irritability come from the fact that you are now consuming fewer carbs than before. Carbs almost immediately turn into sugar when finished, whether the carb is a honey bun or a potato. The body does not care about the difference between healthy or unhealthy food; it just cares that food is coming in. Excess levels of sugar in the blood cause the body to release the hormones dopamine and serotonin, making you calm happy. This hormone release is also why people often fall asleep after consuming a full of carbs. Removing these foods means that the brain will not signal the release of these hormones, and you might feel irritable or moody for a few days.

High-fat diets will increase the estrogen level in the woman's body because estrogen is stored in fat. Estrogen drives your desire for sex, and this is often lost during the first days of ketosis as all of those stored fat cells begin to disappear. When the body has eliminated enough stored fat and has already started functioning properly, the hormone levels will balance it. The estrogen production will return to normal, and your sex drive will reappear.

While these all might seem like good reasons to avoid the keto diet altogether, remember that these side effects are temporary. The beneficial effects of the keto diet are permanent. There are things that you can do to combat the results of the keto flu and the beginning of ketosis to help you get through this period:

- Get a regularly scheduled seven to nine hours of sleep every night
- Engage in gentle exercises like walking, bicycling, or swimming
- Drink plenty of water to stay hydrated
- Add sea salt to your water to help ease muscle cramps. Lemon juice will help mask the saltiness
- Chew gum or suck sugar-free mints

Focusing on the positive benefits of the keto diet may also help you get through ketosis. The keto diet will naturally promote weight loss and assist you with managing your weight. The keto diet will easily incorporate into your everyday lifestyle. Fats and proteins will make you feel full for a more extended period, so you will eventually consume less food. Food cravings will disappear, and hunger will be eliminated. There is no need to count calories on the keto diet unless you are going for a specific weight loss goal. Keto will not slow down your metabolism, so you will continue to lose weight even after the first few weeks on a diet. You will feel more energetic and will be able to better focus on everyday tasks. Your muscles will become stronger and leaner.

Keto flu fades away, and you are left with the positive side effect of the keto diet, which will last your entire lifetime. All bodies are different, and you may not see the same results that your neighbor might enjoy on the same diet plan. But follow the diet, eat the right foods, and you will be successful.

Chapter 2: 11 Reasons Why Women Over 50 Should Try Keto

When the entire ketogenic lifestyle is followed along with dietary changes, it results in the following known benefits:

1. Accelerates Metabolism

As a person ages, it is the rate of metabolism that slows down with time. Metabolism is the sum total of all the processes that are carried out in the body. It consists of the building of new cells and elements, as well as the breaking of the existing agents into other elements. The fat-sourced high energy and release of ketones accelerate the rate of metabolism in the body.

2. Hormones Production

It is said that a woman's body is particularly more sensitive to dietary changes than the male body. It is mainly because there are several hormones that are at play in a woman's body. With a slight change in dietary habits and lifestyle, women can harness more benefits out of their fasting regime. Hormones in women's bodies are not only responsible for regulating the mood and internal body processes, but they also affect other systems in the body. Controlled release of energy and a healthy diet is responsible for maintaining the balance of estrogen and progesterone in the body.

3. Weight Loss

Finally, weight loss is the most promising and obvious advantage of the ketogenic diet. Women over 50 years of age actively seek the keto diet to lose weight. It can reduce two to one and half kilos of weight within a week.

4. Oxidative Stress

There are various chemical reactions that are occurring within the human body as a result of metabolism. These reactions produce millions of products and byproducts. Some chemical reactions produce free radicals, which are highly reactive in nature. When these radicals are left in the body for a longer duration of time, they can oxidize other elements in the cells and mingle with the natural cell cycle, ultimately leading to cell death. The cumulative effect of those free radicals is termed oxidative stress. When this stress increases, it can negatively affect human health. Ketones produced through ketosis work as antioxidants, which remove the free radicals and toxins from the body.

5. Diabetes

Insulin resistance is a condition in which the body resists producing insulin. When the body fails to produce insulin, the pancreatic cells produce more insulin to lower the blood glucose levels. Excessive insulin production over a longer period of time ultimately wears out the pancreatic cells, and they lose the ability to produce necessary insulin levels, thus leading to diabetes. Since intermittent fasting can prevent insulin resistance by naturally lowering blood glucose levels, it also reduces the risks of diabetes. The ketogenic diet controls the insulin levels in the blood, thus prevents the risks of insulin resistance and diabetes.

6. PCOS

Polycystic ovarian syndrome is another common disorder that is prevalent among women of all ages, especially those over 50. PCOS cases are often the result of consistently high levels of insulin in the blood. Therefore, the ketogenic diet, due to its lowering of insulin effect, can treat or prevent PCOS to some extent. It can also control and counter the negative effects of PCOS in women.

7. Cures Cancer

The ketogenic diet also improves the immune system, which helps patients to fight against all sorts of diseases, especially cancer. When the body undergoes ketosis, there is an increased production of lymphocytes that kills the pathogens or agents that may lead to cancer. Several cancer treatments also use this natural immune system to fight against cancerous cells.

8. Inflammation

Inflammation is the swelling of body tissues and organs for any practical reason. In women over the age of 50, inflammation can result from hormonal or electrolyte imbalance. Accumulation of uric acid and high sugar and cholesterol levels may also cause inflammation. Diseases like osteoporosis, or arthritis, which are common among women, also cause inflammation. Similarly, inflammation can also occur in the brain due to Alzheimer's or dementia. In any case, inflammation is always painful and health-damaging. Ketosis can help the body fight against the agents, causing inflammation. It promotes the immune system to increase its productivity. The damaged cells, which cause inflammation in the neighboring area, are then actively removed through autophagy to clean the body and repair it.

9. Athletic Performance with More Energy

When your body burns fat instead of glucose, something magical happens in terms of exercise. Normally, the body will turn towards glucose to fuel workout sessions. This is why some athletes will eat a carby meal hours before they plan to exercise. It provides them with adequate energy to see through a difficult routine. But what sometimes happens is that this energy tapers off in the middle of the workout, bringing performance to a crawl. Almost nobody is a stranger to this effect in the gym. Out of nowhere it seems like you are desperately tired, and you can't push yourself to finish the workout. Your glucose stores have been depleted, and your body needs more to go on. In that scenario we are more likely to end the workout, go home and regroup.

To make up for its dependency on glucose our body can store some of it in the form of glycogen. It is an intermediary between pure close and adipose tissue, usually stored in the liver and muscle cells. Glycogen doesn't get used unless the body requires immediate energy expenditure, like when running after prey in the wild. In the gym, glycogen is most likely to be used up when lifting weights or doing intense cardio sessions. And when all the glycogen is inevitably used up, our bodies feel like they can no longer go on.

In contrast, the process of ketosis provides ample energy that isn't likely to run out like glycogen. Instead of stopping in the middle of the workout you might feel fine throughout. You won't experience any unanticipated drops in blood sugar, which can ruin athletic performance.

This further translates to activities outside of the gym. We are all too familiar with the mid-afternoon crash that happens in the hours between lunch and dinner. Even if we aren't hungry, we start to feel tired and taking a nap in the middle of the office suddenly feels like a good idea. Blood sugar is usually to blame. Even if your body doesn't signal that it is running on empty, it could still be the case that blood sugar is dropping and that you are experience a mild instance of hypoglycemia. The symptoms are feeling tired, irritable or angry with decreased brain function and alertness. Since glucose supply has fallen, your body is compensating by shutting off non-vital activity like mood regulation.

Most will simply reach for another coffee to get over the slump. Others will turn to a sugary or salty snack that is high in refined carbs. It gets them through the rest of the work day until dinner comes around, but the meal can be more detrimental than that. Instead of training your body to eat nutritious, filling food such behavior encourages fluctuations in blood sugar. A small, but energetically dense meal translates to instantaneous energy at the cost of stability. You will continue to experience the same crash unless those eating habits are changed.

Since blood sugar fluctuation doesn't really affect you while on ketosis, the mid-afternoon slump is rare. You can stay productive for eight hours or more during the day and still have more left for doing things outside of work. And you won't feel like dying half way between dinner.

10. Decreased Cardiovascular Risk

Diets high in carbohydrates directly raise bad cholesterol by forming excess triglycerides when excess glucose can't be absorbed. The effect is even worse in individuals with insulin insensitivity problems, wherein glucose has a harder time being metabolized into energy. Going on a keto diet lowers this production of triglycerides due to an influx in carbs.

What's more, keto acts as an anti-inflammatory diet. Using whole foods that are high in antioxidants helps keep long term inflammation down. Inflammation is just as risky to cardiovascular disease as is cholesterol or triglycerides build up.

11. A Cure for Aging

Finally, keto in conjunction with intermittent fasting, (which will be covered later in this book) may help prevent aging. Observational studies both in animal models and humans have found a correlation between calorie restriction and longevity. Some of the oldest people on earth always enjoy a sparse diet, and scientist weren't really sure why. From an non-scientific standpoint it sort of does make sense that eating a little bit will help you live for longer. Your body undergoes less metabolic and digestive stress from eating. A modern equivalent would be a car that is driven often, and with a heavy foot. Frequent hard brakes and acceleration spikes correlate with frequent blood sugar and insulin spikes. Over time a heavy foot will damage the engine and transmission of a car so that its operational life is lower than that of a car driven with more care.

Hints as to why a low-calorie diet makes people live for longer could be found in the ketone body β-hydroxybutyrate, which is present during times of starvation. The same ketone body is also present during prolonged fasts, long exercise sessions, and of course during ketosis. B-hydroxybutyrate can further block certain enzyme histone deacetylases, (HDC's) which are responsible for causing genetic damage in the long term. It could be that low calorie diets, fasting and ketogenic diets all have similar properties which are spurred by the ketone body B-hydroxybutyrate.

Chapter 3: 7 Keto Diet Weight Loss Secrets

Do you feel like you are giving your all to the keto diet but you still aren't seeing the results you want? You are measuring ketones, working out, and counting your macros, but you still aren't losing the weight you want. Here are the most common mistakes that most people make when beginning the keto diet.

1. Too Many Snacks

There are many snacks you can enjoy while following the keto diet, like nuts, avocado, seeds, and cheese. But snacking can be an easy way to get too many calories into the diet while giving your body an easy fuel source besides stored fat. Snacks need to be only used if you frequently hunger between meals. If you aren't extremely hungry, let your body turn to your stored fat for its fuel between meals instead of dietary fat.

2. Not Consuming Enough Fat

The ketogenic diet isn't all about low carbs. It's also about high fats. You need to be getting about 75 percent of your calories from healthy fats, five percent from carbs, and 20 percent from protein. Fat makes you feel fuller longer, so if you eat the correct amount, you will minimize your carb cravings, and this will help you stay in ketosis. This will help your body burn fat faster.

3. Consuming Excessive Calories

You may hear people say you can eat what you want on the keto diet as long as it is high in fat. Even though we want that to be true, it is very misleading. Healthy fats need to make up the biggest part of your diet. If you eat more calories than what you are burning, you will gain weight, no matter what you eat because these excess calories get stored as fat. An average adult only needs about 2,000 calories each day, but this will vary based on many factors like activity level, height, and gender.

4. Consuming a lot of Protein

The biggest mistake that most people make when just beginning the keto diet is consuming too much protein. Excess protein gets converted into glucose in the body called gluconeogenesis. This is a natural process where the body converts the energy from fats and proteins into glucose when glucose isn't available. When following a ketogenic diet, gluconeogenesis happens at different rates to keep body function. Our bodies don't need a lot of carbs, but we do need glucose. You can eat absolute zero carbs, and through gluconeogenesis, your body will convert other substances into glucose to be used as fuel. This is why carbs only make up five percent of your macros. Some parts of our bodies need carbs to survive, like kidney, medulla, and red blood cells. With gluconeogenesis, our bodies make and stores extra glucose as glycogen just in case supplies become too low.

In a normal diet, when carbs are always available, gluconeogenesis happens slowly because the need for glucose is extremely low. Our body runs on glucose and will store excess protein and carbs as fat.

It does take time for our bodies to switch from using glucose to burning fats. Once you are in ketosis, your body will use fat as the main fuel source and will start to store excess protein as glycogen.

5. Not Getting Enough Water

Water is crucial for your body. Water is needed for all your body does, and this includes burning fat. If you don't drink enough water, it can cause your metabolism to slow down, and this can halt your weight loss. Drinking 1800g or one-half gallon every day will help your body burn fat, flush out toxins, and circulate nutrients. When you are just beginning the keto diet, you might need to drink more water since your body will begin to get rid of body fat by flushing it out through urine.

6. Low on Electrolytes

Most people will experience the keto flu when you begin this diet. This happens for two reasons when your body changes from burning carbs to burning fat, your brain might not have enough energy, and this, in turn, can cause grogginess, headaches, and nausea. You could be dehydrated, and your electrolytes might be low since the keto diet causes you to urinate often.

Getting the keto flu is a great sign that you are heading in the right direction. You can lessen these symptoms by drinking more water or taking supplements that will balance your electrolytes.

7. Consuming Hidden Carbs

Many foods look like they are low carb, but they aren't. You can find carbs in salad dressings, sauces, and condiments. Be sure to check nutrition labels before you try new foods to make sure it doesn't have any hidden sugar or carbs. It just takes a few seconds to skim the label, and it might be the difference between whether or not you'll lose weight.

If you have successfully ruled out all of the above, but you still aren't losing weight, you might need to talk with your doctor to make sure you don't have any health problems that could be preventing your weight loss. This can be frustrating, but stick with it, stay positive, and stay in the game. When the keto diet is done correctly, it is one of the best ways to lose weight.

Recipes for Breakfast

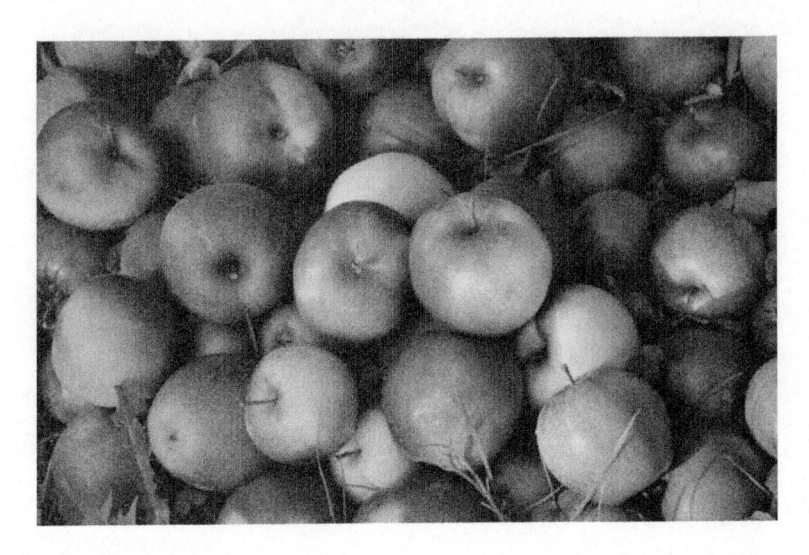

Mayonnaise Waffles

Preparation time: 15 minutes

Cooking time: 10 minutes

Servings: 2

Ingredients:

- 125 ml blanched almond flour
- 30 ml erythritol
- 1.25 ml salt
- 2.5 ml organic baking powder
- 1 large organic egg (separated)
- 60 ml unsweetened almond milk
- 30 ml butter, melted
- 30 ml almond butter, melted
- 2.5 ml organic vanilla extract

Directions:

1. In a large bowl, mix together almond flour, erythritol, baking powder, and salt.
2. In a second clean glass bowl, add the egg white and beat until stiff peaks form. Set aside.
3. In a third bowl, add egg yolks, almond milk, butter, almond butter, and vanilla extract and beat until well combined.
4. Add the flour mixture and mix until smooth.
5. Gently, fold in the whipped egg whites.
6. Preheat the waffle iron and then grease it.
7. Place ½ of the mixture into preheated waffle iron and cook for about 4-5 minutes or until golden-brown.
8. Repeat with the remaining mixture.
9. Serve warm.

Nutrition:
Calories 425 | Net Carbs 4.4 g | Total Fat 38.5 g | Saturated Fat 9.8 g | Cholesterol 124 g | Sodium 134 mg | Total Carbs 9.2 g | Fiber 4.8 g | Sugar 2 g | Protein 6.8 g

Coconut Macadamia Bars

Preparation time: 15 minutes

Cooking time: None

Servings: 6

Ingredients:

- 125 ml macadamia nuts
- 90 ml unsweetened coconut, shredded
- 125 ml almond butter
- 20 stevia drops, preferably Sweet leaf
- 60 ml coconut oil

Directions:

1. Crush the macadamia nuts using hands or in a food processor.
2. Combine coconut oil with the shredded coconut and almond butter in a large-sized mixing bowl. Add the stevia drops and chopped macadamia nuts.
3. Thoroughly mix and pour the prepared batter into a 9x9" baking dish lined with parchment paper.
4. Refrigerate for overnight; slice into desired pieces.
5. Serve and enjoy.

Nutrition:
Calories 324 | Total Fat 32 g | Saturated Fat 13 g | Total Carbs 1.2 g| Dietary Fiber 4 g | Sugars 1.8 g | Protein 5.6 g

Turmeric Muffins

Preparation time: 10 minutes

Cooking time: 23 minutes

Servings: 6

Ingredients:

- 450 ml almond flour
- 125 ml powdered erythritol
- 3 scoops turmeric tonic
- 3 organic eggs
- 250 ml mayonnaise
- 2.5 ml organic vanilla extract
- 12.5 ml organic baking powder

Directions:

1. Preheat your oven to 176 C.
2. Line a 1450 ml muffin tin with paper liners.
3. In a large bowl, add flour, erythritol, turmeric tonic, and baking powder, and mix well.
4. Add the eggs, mayonnaise, and vanilla extract, and beat until well combined.
5. Place the mixture into the prepared muffin cups evenly.
6. Bake for approximately 20–23 minutes or until a toothpick inserted in the center comes out clean.
7. Remove the muffin tin from oven and place onto a wire rack to cool for about 10 minutes.
8. Carefully invert the muffins onto the wire rack to cool completely before serving.

Nutrition:
Calories 516 | Net Carbs 3.9 g | Total Fat 48.9 g | Saturated Fat 6 g | Cholesterol 95 mg | Sodium 272 mg | Total Carbs 8 g | Fiber 4.1 g | Sugar 1.9 g | Protein 2.8 g

Bacon Avocado Bombs

Preparation time: 10 minutes

Cooking time: 1 hour

Servings: 4

Ingredients:

- 2 avocados
- 75 ml shredded Cheddar
- 8 slices bacon

Directions:

1. Boil the egg for 6 minutes.
2. Add in the cold water and allow to cool, Peel the eggs.
3. A bit at a time, enlarge the stone-hole in the avocado to fit the egg.
4. Then put it back together with the egg inside.
5. Wrap the egg avocado in streaky bacon tightly,
6. Heat the oil in a deep-fryer to 176 C.
7. With a spoon, with care, lower the avocado egg in the fryer and fry until bacon is golden brown.
8. Add a splash of warm water to the smoked chipotle chili honey in a bowl and stir to smoothen.
9. Use a pastry brush to glaze the bacon with the honey.
10. Allow to cool and cut along the fault line in the avocado.
11. Season the egg with a little salt and pepper.

Nutrition: Calories 117 | Carbs 0.4 g | Fat 10.1 g | Protein 7.3 g

Tofu & Mushroom Muffins

Preparation time: 15 minutes

Cooking time: 30 minutes

Servings: 6

Ingredients:

- 5 ml olive oil
- 375 ml fresh mushrooms, chopped
- 1 scallion, chopped
- 5 ml garlic, minced
- 5 ml fresh rosemary, minced
- Freshly ground black pepper, to taste
- 1 (350gms) package lite firm silken tofu, drained
- 60 ml unsweetened almond milk
- 30 ml Parmesan cheese, grated
- 15 ml arrowroot starch
- 5 ml butter, softened
- 1.25 ml ground turmeric

Directions:

1. Preheat your oven to 190 C.
2. Grease a 1450 ml muffin tin.
3. In a non-stick skillet, heat the oil over medium heat and sauté the scallion and garlic for about 1 minute.
4. Add the mushrooms and sauté for about 5–7 minutes.
5. Stir in the rosemary and black pepper and remove from the heat.
6. Set aside to cool slightly.
7. In a food processor, add the tofu and remaining ingredients and pulse until smooth.
8. Transfer the tofu mixture into a large bowl.
9. Fold in the mushroom mixture.

10. Place the mixture into the prepared muffin cups evenly.
11. Bake for approximately 20–22 minutes or until a toothpick inserted in the center comes out clean.
12. Remove the muffin pan from the oven and place onto a wire rack to cool for about 10 minutes.
13. Carefully invert the muffins onto wire rack and serve warm.

Nutrition:
Calories 63 | Net Carbs 2.3 g | Total Fat 3.6 g | Saturated Fat 1 g | Total Carbs 2.8 g | Fiber 0.5 g | Sugar 1.1 g | Protein 5.4 g

---

Chicken, Bacon, Avocado Caesar Salad

Preparation time: 10 minutes

Cooking time: None

Servings: 4

Ingredients:

- 1 chicken breast, pre-cooked or grilled, sliced into small bite sized slices
- 1 avocado, ripe, sliced in half, twist and discard the pit, remove the shell and slice into approximately 1" slices.
- Creamy Caesar dressing (approximately 45 ml per salad)
- 250 ml bacon, pre-cooked, crumbled

Directions:

1. Combine the chicken breast with avocado slices and crumbled bacon between two large sized bowls.
2. Top with a few spoonsful of the Creamy Caesar dressing; lightly toss the ingredients.
3. Serve immediately and enjoy.

Nutrition:
Calories 322 | Total Fat 30 g | Saturated Fat 8.6 g | Total Carbs 5 g | Dietary Fiber 3.4 g | Sugars 0.9 g | Protein 9.2 g

---

Shrimp and Olives Pan

Preparation time: 5 minutes

Cooking time: 15 minutes

Servings: 4

Ingredients:

- 450g shrimp, peeled and deveined
- 10 ml sweet paprika
- 250 ml black olives, pitted and halved
- 15 ml olive oil
- 125 ml kalamata olives, pitted and halved
- Salt and black pepper to the taste
- 2 spring onions, chopped
- 125 ml heavy cream

Directions:

1. Heat up a pan with the oil over medium heat, add the onions, toss and cook for 2 minutes.
2. Add the shrimp and the other ingredients except the cream, toss and cook for 4 minutes more.
3. Add the cream, toss, cook over medium heat for another 4 minutes.
4. Divide everything between plates and serve for breakfast.

Nutrition:
Calories 263 | Fat 14.8 g | Fiber 1.7 g | Carbs 5.5 g | Protein 26.7 g

Baked Eggs

Preparation time: 10 minutes

Cooking time: 12 minutes

Servings: 4

Ingredients:

- 60 ml half-and-half
- 4 organic eggs
- 15gms Gruyere cheese, shredded
- Salt and ground black pepper, to taste
- 20 ml fresh chives, minced

Directions:

1. Preheat your oven to 190 C.
2. Grease 4 ramekins.
3. In the bottom of each prepared ramekin, place 15 ml of the heavy cream.
4. Carefully, crack 1 egg into each ramekin and sprinkle with the cheese, followed by salt, black pepper, and chives.
5. Bake for approximately 8–12 minutes until the desired doneness of the eggs.
6. Serve hot.

Nutrition:
Calories 97 | Net Carbs 1 g | Total Fat 7.3 g | Saturated Fat 3.1 g | Cholesterol 173 mg | Sodium 118 mg | Total Carbs 1 g | Fiber 0 g | Sugar 0.4 g | Protein 7.1 g

---

Crêpes with Lemon-Buttery Syrup

Preparation time: 15 minutes

Cooking time: 20 minutes

Servings: 6

Ingredients:

- 170gms mascarpone cheese, softened
- 6 eggs
- 22.5 ml granulated swerve
- 60 ml almond flour
- 5 ml baking soda
- 5 ml baking powder

For the Syrup:

- 175 ml of water
- 30 ml lemon juice
- 15 ml butter
- 175 ml swerve, powdered
- 15 ml vanilla extract
- 2.5 ml xanthan gum

Directions:

1. With the use of an electric mixer, mix all crepes ingredients until well incorporated.
2. Use melted butter to grease a frying pan and set over medium heat; cook the crepes.
3. Flip over and cook the other side for a further 2 minutes; repeat the remaining batter.
4. Put the crepes on a plate.
5. In the same pan, mix swerve, butter and water; simmer for 6 minutes as you stir.

6. Transfer the mixture to a blender and a 1.25 ml of xanthan gum and vanilla extract and mix well.
7. Place in the remaining 1.25 ml of xanthan gum and allow to sit until the syrup is thick.

Nutrition:
Calories 312 | Fat 11.5 g | Fiber 3.8 g | Carbs 2.4 g | Protein 5.1 g

Yogurt Waffles

Preparation time: 15 minutes

Cooking time: 25 minutes

Servings: 5

Ingredients:

- 125 ml golden flax seeds meal
- 125 ml plus 45 ml almond flour
- 15-22.5 ml granulated Erythritol
- 15 ml unsweetened vanilla whey protein powder
- 1.25 ml baking soda
- 2.5 ml organic baking powder
- 1.25 ml xanthan gum
- Salt, as required
- 1 large organic egg, white and yolk separated
- 1 organic whole egg
- 30 ml unsweetened almond milk
- 22.5 ml unsalted butter
- 85 grams plain Greek yogurt

Directions:

1. Preheat the waffle iron and then grease it.
2. In a large bowl, add the flour, Erythritol, protein powder, baking soda, baking powder, xanthan gum, salt, and mix until well combined.
3. In another bowl or container, put in the egg white and beat until stiff peaks form.
4. In a third bowl, add two egg yolks, whole egg, almond milk, butter, yogurt, and beat until well combined.
5. Place egg mixture into the bowl of the flour mixture and mix until well combined.

6. Gently, fold in the beaten egg whites.
7. Place 60 ml of the mixture into preheated waffle iron and cook for about 4–5 minutes or until golden brown.
8. Repeat with the remaining mixture.
9. Serve warm.

Nutrition:
Calories 265 | Fat 11.5 g | Fiber 9.5 g | Carbs 5.2 g | Protein 7.5 g

---

Bacon Omelet

Preparation time: 15 minutes

Cooking time: 15 minutes

Servings: 2

Ingredients:

- 4 large organic eggs
- 15 ml fresh chives, minced
- Salt and ground black pepper, to taste
- 4 bacon slices
- 15 ml unsalted butter
- 55g cheddar cheese, shredded

Directions:

1. In a bowl, add the eggs, chives, salt, and black pepper, and beat until well combined.
2. Heat a non-stick frying pan over medium-high heat and cook the bacon slices for about 8–10 minutes.
3. Place the bacon onto a paper towel-lined plate to drain. Then chop the bacon slices.
4. With paper towels, wipe out the frying pan.
5. In the same frying pan, melt the butter over medium-low heat and cook the egg mixture for about 2 minutes.
6. Carefully flip the omelet and top with chopped bacon.
7. Cook for 1–2 minutes or until desired doneness of eggs.
8. Remove from heat and immediately place the cheese in the center of omelet.
9. Fold the edges of omelet over cheese and cut into 2 portions.
10. Serve immediately.

Nutrition:
Calories 622 | Net Carbs 2 g | Total Fat 49.3 g | Saturated Fat 20.7 g | Cholesterol 481 mg | Total Carbs 2 g | Fiber 0 g | Sugar 1 g | Protein 41.2 g

Bell Pepper Frittata

Preparation time: 15 minutes

Cooking time: 10 minutes

Servings: 6

Ingredients:

- 8 organic eggs
- 15 ml fresh cilantro, chopped
- 15 ml fresh basil, chopped
- 1.25 ml red pepper flakes, crushed
- Salt and ground black pepper, to taste
- 30 ml unsalted butter
- 1 bunch scallions, chopped
- 250 ml bell pepper, seeded and sliced thinly
- 125 ml goat cheese, crumbled

Directions:

1. Preheat the broiler of oven.
2. Arrange a rack in upper third of the oven.
3. In a bowl, add the eggs, fresh herbs, red pepper flakes, salt, and black pepper, and beat well.
4. In an ovenproof skillet, melt the butter over medium heat and sauté the scallion and bell pepper for about 1 minute.
5. Add the egg mixture over bell pepper mixture evenly and lift the edges to let the egg mixture flow underneath and cook for about 2–3 minutes.
6. Place the cheese on top in the form of dots.
7. Now, transfer the skillet under broiler and broil for about 2–3 minutes.
8. Remove from the oven and set aside for about 5 minutes before serving.

9. Cut the frittata into desired-sized slices and serve.

Nutrition:
Calories 183 | Net Carbs 0 g | Total Fat 14.4 g | Saturated Fat 7.3 g | Cholesterol 248 mg Sodium 338 mg | Total Carbs 2.3 g | Fiber 0.4 g | Sugar 1 g | Protein 11.7 g

---

Recipes for Lunch

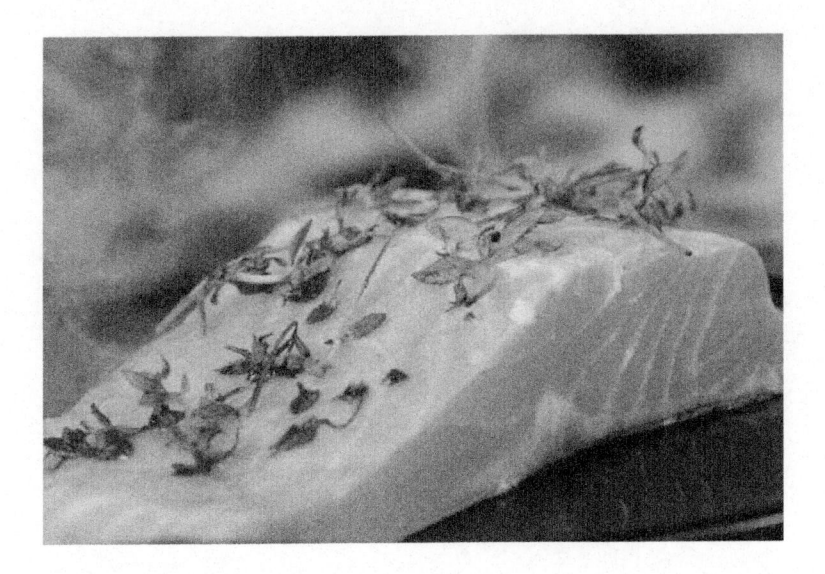

Broccoli and Turkey Dish

Preparation Time: 5 Minutes

Cooking Time: 15 Minutes

Servings: 2

Ingredients:

- 1.25 ml red pepper flakes
- 15 ml olive oil
- 5 ml soy sauce
- 115g broccoli florets
- 115g cauliflower florets, riced
- 115g ground turkey

Directions:

1. Bring out a skillet pan, place it over medium heat.
2. Add olive oil and when hot, add beef. Crumble it and cook for 8 minutes until no longer pink.
3. Then add broccoli florets and riced cauliflower. Stir well, drizzle with soy sauce and sesame oil, season with salt, black pepper, and red pepper flakes.
4. Continue cooking for 5 minutes until vegetables have been thoroughly cooked.

Nutrition: Calories: 120.3 Fats: 8.3g Protein: 8.4g Net Carb: 2g Fiber: 1g

Zucchini Sushi

Preparation Time: 20 Minutes

Cooking Time: 0 Minutes

Servings: 2

Ingredients:

- 2 zucchinis
- 115g cream cheese
- 5 ml Sriracha hot sauce
- 5 ml lime juice
- 250 ml lump crab meat
- 1/2 carrot
- 1/2 avocado
- 1/2 cucumber
- 5 ml toasted sesame seeds

Directions:

1. Slice each zucchini into thin flat strips. Put aside.
2. Combine cream cheese, sriracha, and lime juice in a medium-sized cup.
3. Place two slices of zucchini horizontally flat on a cutting board.
4. Place a lean layer of cream cheese over it, then top the left with a slice of lobster, carrot, avocado, and cucumber.
5. Roll up zucchini. Serve with sesame seeds.

Nutrition: Calories: 450   Carbohydrates: 23g   Fat: 25g   Protein: 35g

Easy Mayo Salmon

Preparation Time: 5 Minutes

Cooking Time: 10 Minutes

Servings: 2

Ingredients:

- 2 salmon fillets
- 60 ml mayonnaise

Directions:

1. Turn on the panini press, spray it with oil, and let it preheat.
2. Spread 15 ml of mayonnaise on each side of the salmon, place them on Panini press pan, shut with a lid, and cook for 7 to 10 minutes until the salmon has cooked to the desired level.

Nutrition: Calories: 132.7 Fats: 11.1g Protein: 8g Net Carb: 0.3g

Caprese Zoodles

Preparation Time: 15 Minutes

Cooking Time: 0 Minutes

Servings: 2

Ingredients:

- 2 zucchinis
- 15 ml extra-virgin olive oil
- Kosher salt
- Ground black pepper
- 250 ml cherry tomatoes halved
- 250 ml mozzarella balls
- 30 ml basil leaves
- 15 ml balsamic vinegar

Directions:

1. Creating zoodles out of zucchini using a spiralizer.
2. Mix the zoodles, olive oil, salt, and pepper. Marinate for 15 minutes.
3. Put the tomatoes, mozzarella, and basil and toss.
4. Drizzle, and drink with balsamic vinegar.

Nutrition: Calories: 417 Carbohydrates: 11g Fat: 24g Protein: 36g

Zesty Avocado and Lettuce Salad

Preparation Time: 5 Minutes

Cooking Time: 0 Minutes

Servings: 2

Ingredients:

- ½ of a lime, juiced
- 1 avocado, pitted, sliced
- 30 ml olive oil
- 115g chopped lettuce
- 60 ml chopped chives

Directions:

1. In a small bowl, add oil, lime juice, salt, and black pepper, stir until mixed, and then slowly mix oil until the dressing is combined.
2. Bring out a large bowl, add avocado, lettuce, and chives, and then toss gently.
3. Drizzle with dressing, toss until well coated. Serve.

Nutrition: Calories: 125.7 Fats: 11g Protein: 1.3g Net Carb: 1.7g Fiber: 3.7g

---

Keto Buffalo Chicken Empanadas

Preparation Time: 20 Minutes

Cooking Time: 30 Minutes

Servings: 2

Ingredients:

- For the empanada dough
- 175 ml mozzarella cheese
- 30g cream cheese
- 1 whisked egg
- 250 ml almond flour
- For the buffalo chicken filling
- 250 ml shredded chicken
- 15 ml butter
- 60 ml Hot Sauce

Directions:

1. Warm up the oven to 215 C.
2. Microwave the cheese & cream cheese within one minute.
3. Stir the flour and egg into the dish.
4. In another bowl, combine the chicken with sauce and set aside.
5. Cover a flat surface with plastic wrap and sprinkle with almond flour.
6. Grease a rolling pin, press the dough flat.
7. Make the circle shapes out of this dough with a lid.
8. Portion out spoonful of filling into these dough circles.
9. Fold the other half over to close up into half-moon shapes.
10. Bake within 9 minutes. Serve.

Nutrition: Net carbohydrates: 20g   Fiber: 0g   Fat: 96g   Protein: 74g   Calories: 1217kcal

Pepperoni and Cheddar Stromboli

Preparation Time: 15 Minutes

Cooking Time: 20 Minutes

Servings: 2

Ingredients:

- 310 ml mozzarella cheese
- 60 ml almond flour
- 45 ml coconut flour
- 5 ml Italian seasoning
- 1 egg
- 170g deli ham
- 55g pepperoni
- 115g cheddar cheese
- 15 ml butter
- 1.45L salad greens

Directions:

1. Warm up the oven to 204°C.
2. Melt the mozzarella.
3. Mix flours & Italian seasoning in a separate bowl.
4. Dump in the melty cheese and mix with pepper and salt.
5. Stir in the egg and process the dough.
6. Pour it onto that prepared baking tray.
7. Roll out the dough. Cut slits that mark out 4 equal rectangles.
8. Put the ham and cheese, then brush with butter and close up.
9. Bake within 17 minutes. Slice and serve.

Nutrition: Net carbohydrates: 20g Fiber: 0g Fat: 13g Protein: 11g Calories: 240kcal

Veggie, Bacon, and Egg Dish

Preparation Time: 5 Minutes

Cooking Time: 5 Minutes

Servings: 2

Ingredients:

- 60 ml mayonnaise
- 2 eggs, boiled, sliced
- 115g spinach
- 4 slices of bacon, chopped

Directions:

1. Heat a skillet pan over medium heat, add bacon, and cook for 5 minutes until browned.
2. In a salad bowl, add spinach, top with bacon and eggs, and drizzle with mayonnaise.
3. Toss until well mixed and then serve.

Nutrition: Calories: 181.5 Fats: 16.7g Protein: 7.3g Net Carb: 0.2g Fiber: 0.3g

Hot Spicy Chicken

Preparation Time: 5 Minutes

Cooking Time: 25 Minutes

Servings: 2

Ingredients:

- 3.75 ml fennel seeds, ground
- 1.25 ml smoked paprika
- 2.5 ml hot paprika
- 2.5 ml minced garlic
- 2 chicken thighs, boneless

Directions:

1. Preheat the oven to 162°C.
2. To prepare the spice mix, add all the ingredients in a small bowl except for chicken. Stir until well mixed.
3. Brush the mixture on all sides of the chicken, rub it well into the meat, then place the chicken onto a baking sheet.
4. Roast for 15 to 25 minutes until thoroughly cooked, basting every 10 minutes with the drippings.

Nutrition: Calories: 102.3 Fats: 8g Protein: 7.2g Net Carb: 0.3g Fiber: 0.3g

Keto Teriyaki Chicken

Preparation Time: 5 Minutes

Cooking Time: 18 Minutes

Servings: 2

Ingredients:

- 15 ml olive oil
- 15 ml swerve sweetener
- 2 chicken thighs, boneless
- 30 ml soy sauce

Directions:

1. Heat a skillet pan over medium heat.
2. Add oil and when hot, add chicken thighs. Cook for 5 minutes per side until seared.
3. Then sprinkle sugar over chicken thighs, drizzle with soy sauce, and bring the sauce to boil.
4. Switch heat to medium-low level, continue cooking for 3 minutes until chicken is evenly glazed, and then transfer to a plate.
5. Serve chicken with cauliflower rice.

Nutrition: Calories: 150 Fats: 9g Protein: 17.3g Net Carb: 0g Fiber: 0g

California Burger Bowls

Preparation Time: 15 Minutes

Cooking Time: 20 Minutes

Servings: 2

Ingredients:

For the dressing:

- 60 ml extra-virgin olive oil
- 45 ml balsamic vinegar
- 22.5 ml Dijon mustard
- 5 ml honey
- 1/2 clove garlic
- Kosher salt
- Ground black pepper

For the burger:

- 225g grass-fed organic ground beef
- 2.5 ml Worcestershire sauce
- 1.25 ml chili powder
- 1.25 ml onion powder
- Kosher salt
- Ground black pepper
- 1/2 package butterhead lettuce
- 1/2 medium red onion
- 1/2 avocado
- 1 tomato

Directions:

1. To make the dressing, mix the dressing items in a medium bowl.

2. To make burgers, combine beef and Worcestershire sauce, chili powder, and onion powder in another large bowl. Put pepper and salt, mix.
3. Form into four patties.
4. Grill the onions within 3 minutes each. Remove and detach burgers from the grill pan. Cook within 4 minutes per side.
5. To plate, put lettuce in a large bowl with 1/2 the dressing. Finish with a patty burger, grilled onions, 1/4 slices of avocado, and tomatoes. Serve.

Nutrition: Calories: 407 Carbohydrates: 33g Fat: 19g Protein: 26g

Parmesan Brussels Sprouts Salad

Preparation Time: 15 Minutes

Cooking Time: 25 Minutes

Servings: 2

Ingredients:

- 30 ml extra-virgin olive oil
- 30 ml lemon juice
- 60 ml parsley
- Kosher salt
- Ground black pepper
- 225g Brussels sprouts
- 60 ml toasted almonds
- 60 ml pomegranate seeds
- Shaved Parmesan

Directions:

1. Mix olive oil, lemon juice, parsley, 10 ml of salt, and 5 ml of pepper.
2. Add the Brussels sprouts in and toss.
3. Let sit before serving within 20 minutes and up to 4 hours.
4. Fold in almonds and pomegranate seeds and garnish with a rasped parmesan. Serve.

Nutrition: Calories: 130 Carbohydrates: 8g Fat: 9g Protein: 4g

Dinner Recipes

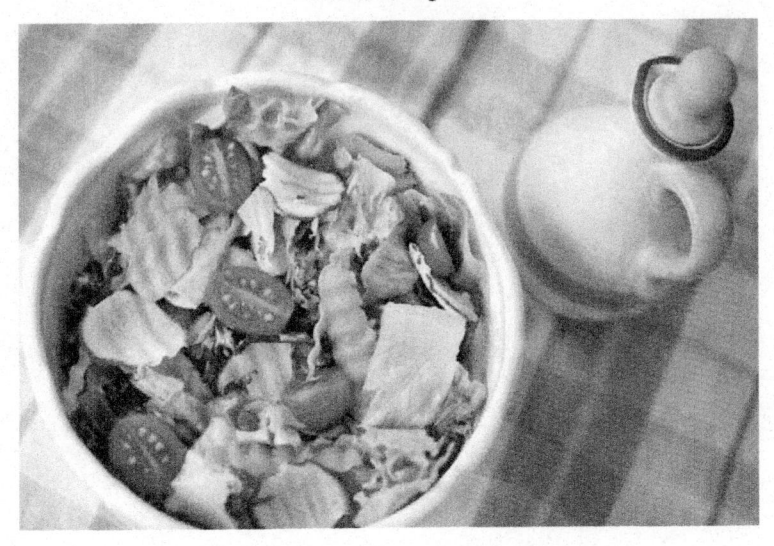

Broccoli and Chicken Casserole

Preparation Time: 15 minutes

Cooking Time: 10 minutes

Servings: 4

Ingredients:

- 680g chicken breast
- 225g softened cream cheese
- 125 ml heavy cream
- 5 ml powdered garlic
- 5 ml powdered onion
- 2.5 ml. salt
- 2.5 ml. pepper
- 450 ml broccoli florets
- 250 ml mozzarella
- 250 ml parmesan

Directions:

1. Heat the oven to a temperature of 204°C.
2. Combine the cream cheese with pepper and salt. Stir in the cubed chicken.
3. Put in the baking dish. Put the broccoli into the chicken-cheese mixture.
4. Top the dish with cheese, bake for about 26 minutes and remove. Take off the foil and bake again for 10 minutes. Serve.

Nutrition: Calories: 391, Fat: 25 g, Protein: 21 g, Net carbs: 20 g, Fiber: 0g

Crispy Peanut Tofu and Cauliflower Rice Stir-Fry

Preparation Time: 15 minutes

Cooking Time: 1 hour

Servings: 4

Ingredients:

- 340g tofu
- 15 ml toasted sesame oil
- 2 cloves minced garlic
- 1 cauliflower head

Sauce:

- 22.5 ml Toasted sesame oil
- 2.5 ml. chili garlic sauce
- 37.5 ml peanut butter
- 60 ml low sodium soy sauce
- 125 ml light brown sugar

Directions:

1. Heat the oven to 204°C. Cube the tofu.
2. Bake for 25 minutes and cool.
3. Combine the sauce ingredients. Put the tofu in the sauce and stir. Leave for 15 minutes.
4. Cook the veggies on a bit of sesame oil and soy sauce. Set it aside.
5. Grab the tofu and put it on the pan. Stir, then set aside.
6. Steam the cauliflower rice for 5 to 8 minutes. Add some sauce and stir.
7. Add up the ingredients. Put the cauliflower rice with the veggies and tofu. Serve.

Nutrition: Calories: 524, Fat: 34 g, Protein: 25 g, Carbs: 39 g

Chicken Schnitzel

Preparation Time: 15 minutes

Cooking Time: 15 minutes

Servings: 3

Ingredients:

- 450g chicken breast
- 125 ml almond flour
- 1 egg
- 7.5 ml powdered garlic
- 7.5 ml powdered onion
- Keto-Safe Oil

Directions:

1. Combine the garlic powder, flour, and onion in a bowl. Separately, beat the egg.
2. With a mallet, 450g out the chicken. Put the chicken in the egg mixture. Then roll well through the flour.
3. Take a deep-frying pan and Heat the oil to medium-high temperature.
4. Add chicken in batches. Fry. Pat dry and serve.

Nutrition: Calories: 541, Fat: 17 g, Protein: 61 g, Net carbs: 32 g, Fiber: 0 g

Mexican Shredded Beef

Preparation Time: 10 minutes

Cooking Time: 7 hours and 15 minutes

Servings: 8

Ingredients:

- 1500g Beef short ribs, grass-fed
- 30 ml Minced garlic
- 10 ml Ground turmeric
- 5 ml Salt
- 2.5 ml Ground black pepper
- 10 ml Ground cumin
- 10 ml Ground coriander
- 5 ml Chipotle powder
- 125 ml Water
- 250 ml Cilantro stems, chopped

Directions:

1. Place salt in a small bowl, add black pepper, cumin, coriander, chipotle powder, and stir until mixed.
2. Place ribs into the slow cooker, sprinkle well with the prepared spice mixture, and then top with minced garlic and cilantro stems.
3. Switch on the slow cooker, pour in water, then cover with the lid and cook for 6 to 7 hours over low heat setting or until tender.
4. Then, pour the sauce into a small saucepan and cook for 10 to 15 minutes or until reduced by half.
5. Return the sauce into the slow cooker, pull apart the meat and toss until well mixed.
6. Portion out beef into eight glass meal prep containers, then cover with a lid and store in the refrigerator for up to 5 days or freeze for up to 2 months.

7. When ready to serve, reheat the beef in its glass container in the microwave for 1 to 2 minutes or until hot.

Nutrition: Calories: 656; Fat: 48.5 g; Protein: 50.2 g; Net Carbs: 1 g; Fiber: 0.4 g

Creamy Chicken Bake

Preparation Time: 15 minutes

Cooking Time: 1 hour 10 minutes

Servings: 6

Ingredients:

- 75 ml unsalted butter
- 2 onions
- 3 garlic cloves
- 5 ml tarragon
- 225g cream cheese
- 250 ml chicken broth
- 30 ml lemon juice
- 125 ml heavy cream
- 12.5 ml. Herbs de Provence
- Salt
- Ground black pepper
- 4 grass-fed chicken breasts

Directions:

1. Heat the oven to 175°C.
2. Cook the onion, garlic, and tarragon for 4–5 minutes. Transfer.
3. Cook the cream cheese, 125 ml of broth, and lemon juice for 3–4 minutes.
4. Stir in the cream, herbs de Provence, salt, and black pepper, remove.
5. Pour remaining broth and chicken breast plus the cream mixture. Bake for 45–60 minutes. Serve.

Nutrition: Calories: 729, Total Fat: 52.8 g, Protein: 55.8 g, Net Carbs: 5.6 g, Sugar: 2 g

Beef Stew

Preparation Time: 5 minutes

Cooking Time: 8 hours and 5 minutes

Servings: 4

Ingredients:

- 1500g Beef, grass-fed, diced
- 3 Stalks celery, chopped
- 1 Leek, white part only
- 425g. Diced tomatoes
- 60 ml Spinach leaves, fresh
- 3 Carrots, chopped into large rounds
- 15 ml Chopped ginger
- 7.5 ml Minced garlic
- 7.5 ml. Salt
- 3.75 ml Ground black pepper
- 10 ml Dried rosemary
- 10 ml Dried thyme
- 10 ml Dried oregano
- 30 ml Apple cider vinegar
- 30 ml Avocado oil
- 375 ml Beef broth, grass-fed

Directions:

1. Take a frying pan, place it over medium heat, add oil and when hot, add beef and cook for 3 to 5 minutes or until light brown.
2. Transfer beef into a slow cooker, add remaining ingredients, except for spinach, and stir until mixed.
3. Switch on the slow cooker, shut it with a lid and cook for 5 to 8 hours at a low heat setting until thoroughly cooked.

4. When beef cooking is about to finish, place spinach in a heatproof bowl, cover with plastic wrap, and microwave for 2 minutes until steamed.
5. When beef is cooked, taste to adjust seasoning, add spinach and stir until just mixed and let cool.
6. Divide beef evenly between four glass containers, then cover with lid and store in the refrigerator for up to 5 days or freeze for up to 2 months.
7. When ready to serve, thaw the stew at room temperature and then reheat the beef stew in its glass container in the microwave for 2 to 3 minutes or until hot.
8. Serve the stew with cauliflower rice.

Nutrition: Calories: 553; Fat: 36.9 g; Protein: 175 g; Net Carbs: 4.8 g; Fiber: 1.6 g

Baked Jerked Chicken

Preparation Time: 20 minutes

Cooking Time: 1 hour and 30 minutes

Servings: 4

Ingredients:

- 910g chicken thighs
- 30 ml Olive Oil
- 30 ml Apple Cider Vinegar
- 5 ml salt
- 5 ml powdered onion
- 2.5 ml. garlic
- 2.5 ml. nutmeg
- 2.5 ml. pepper
- 2.5 ml. powdered ginger
- 2.5 ml. powdered cayenne
- 1.25 ml cinnamon
- 1.25 ml dried thyme

Directions:

1. Mix all the ingredients, excluding the chicken. Stir in the prepared chicken pieces. Stir well.
2. Marinade for 4 hours. Heat the oven to a temperature of 190°C.
3. Cook for 1.25 hours. Adjust to broil chicken for 4 minutes. Serve.

Nutrition: Calories: 185, Fat: 12 g Protein: 16 g, Net Carbs: 4 g Fiber: 0 g

Simple Keto Fried Chicken

Preparation Time: 15 minutes

Cooking Time: 45 minutes

Servings: 4

Ingredients:

- 4 boneless chicken thighs
- Frying oil
- 2 eggs
- 30 ml heavy whipping cream

Breading:

- 150 ml grated parmesan cheese
- 150 ml blanched almond flour
- 5 ml salt
- 2.5 ml. black pepper
- 2.5 ml. cayenne
- 2.5 ml. paprika

Directions:

1. Beat the eggs and heavy cream. Separately, mix all the breading ingredients. Set aside.
2. Cut the chicken thigh into 3 even pieces.
3. Dip the chicken in the bread first before dipping it in the egg wash and then finally, dipping it in the breading again. Fry chicken for 5 minutes. Pat dry the chicken. Serve.

Nutrition: Calories: 304, Fat: 15 g, Protein: 30 g, Carbs: 12 g

Salmon & Shrimp Stew

Preparation Time: 20 minutes

Cooking Time: 25 minutes

Servings: 6

Ingredients:

- 30 ml coconut oil
- 125 ml onion
- 2 garlic cloves
- 1 Serrano pepper
- 5 ml smoked paprika
- 450 ml sliced tomatoes
- 4 cups chicken broth
- 450g salmon fillets
- 450g shrimp
- 30 ml lime juice
- Salt
- Ground black pepper
- 45 ml parsley

Directions:

1. Sauté the onion for 5–6 minutes. Add the garlic, Serrano pepper, and paprika. Add the tomatoes and broth, then boil. Simmer for 5 minutes. Add the salmon and simmer again for 3–4 minutes.
2. Put in the shrimp, then cook for 4–5 minutes. Mix in lemon juice, salt, and black pepper, and remove. Serve with parsley.

Nutrition: Calories: 247, Fiber: 1.2 g, Sugar: 2.1 g, Protein: 32.7 g, Net Carbs: 3.9 g

Sausage Stuffed Zucchini Boats

Preparation Time: 10 minutes

Cooking Time: 30 minutes

Servings: 4

Ingredients:

- 4 Medium zucchini
- 450g Ground Italian pork sausage, pastured
- 1 2.5 ml. Sea salt
- 75 ml Medium white onion, peeled, diced
- 15 ml Minced garlic
- 5 ml Italian seasoning
- 410g. Diced tomatoes
- 75 ml Grated parmesan cheese, full-fat
- 30 ml Avocado oil, divided
- 250 ml Mozzarella cheese, full-fat, shredded

Directions:

1. Set the oven to 204°C and let preheat.
2. Meanwhile, cut each zucchini in half, lengthwise, then make a well in the center by scooping out the centers by using a spoon.
3. Take a baking sheet, line it with a parchment sheet, place zucchini halves on it, cut side up, drizzle with 15 ml oil, and season with salt.
4. Place the baking sheet into the oven and bake for 15 to 20 minutes or until soft.
5. Meanwhile, take a large skillet pan, place it over medium-high heat, add remaining oil and when hot, add onions and cook for 10 minutes until nicely brown.
6. Add sausage, stir well and cook for 5 minutes or until brown.
7. Then, move sausage to one side of the pan, add garlic to the other side, cook for 1 minute or until fragrant, and then mix into the sausage.

8. Remove the pan from the heat, season sausage with Italian seasoning, add tomatoes and parmesan cheese, stir well and taste to adjust seasoning.
9. When zucchini halves are roasted, pat dry with paper towels, then stuff with sausage mixture.
10. Top stuffed zucchini with mozzarella cheese and bake for 5 to 10 minutes or until cheese melts, and the top is nicely golden brown.
11. Let zucchini boats cool down, then wrap each zucchini boat with aluminum foil and freeze in the freezer.
12. When ready to serve, thaw the zucchini boat and reheat at 175°C for 3 to 4 minutes until hot.

Nutrition: Calories: 582; Fat: 44 g; Protein: 29 g; Net Carbs: 11 g; Fiber: 3 g

Balsamic Steaks

Preparation Time: 3 hours and 10 minutes

Cooking Time: 10 minutes

Servings: 4

Ingredients:

- 4 Sirloin steaks, each about 225g, grass-fed
- 15 ml Butter, unsalted

For the marinade:

- 2.5 ml Garlic powder
- 60 ml Coconut aminos
- 2.5 ml Ground black pepper
- 60 ml Avocado oil
- 30 ml Balsamic vinegar
- 5 ml Italian seasoning
- 5 ml Sea salt

Directions:

1. Place all the ingredients for the marinade in a bowl, whisk until well combined, and then pour the mixture into a large freezer bag.
2. Add steaks into the bag, seal the bag, then turn it upside side or until steaks are coated with the marinade and place it in the refrigerator for 3 hours.
3. When ready to cook, set the oven to 204°C and let preheat.
4. In the meantime, take out steaks from the refrigerator and let them rest at room temperature.
5. Then, take a large skillet pan, place it over medium heat, add butter and when it melts, add steaks in a single layer and cook for 2 minutes per side or until seared.
6. Transfer the pan into the oven and bake the stakes for 3 to 6 minutes or until cooked to desired doneness, such as 3 minutes or 45°C for medium-rare doneness, 4 minutes or 60CF for medium doneness, 5

minutes or 65°C for medium-well doneness, and 6 minutes or 70°C for a well-done steak.

7. Transfer the steaks to a plate, let them rest for 5 minutes, and cut into slices.
8. Then transfer steaks into a freezer bag and store in the freezer for up to 3 months.
9. When ready to serve, reheat the steak slices into a hot skillet pan until warm through.

Nutrition: Calories: 450; Fat: 24 g; Protein: 49 g; Net Carbs: 5 g; Fiber: 0 g

Dessert Recipes

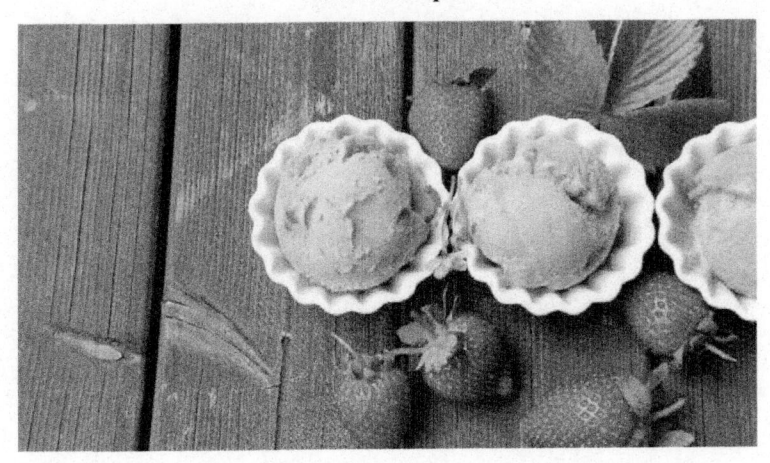

Keto Sorbet

Preparation time: 20 minutes

Cooking time: 0 minutes

Servings: 2

Ingredients:

- 150 ml lemon
- 250 ml frozen blackberries
- 250 ml frozen raspberries
- 15 ml stevia
- 250 ml water

Directions:

1. Place lemon, blackberries, raspberries, stevia, and water in a blender, and blend until smooth. Keep in the freezer to harden. Serve chilled.

Nutrition: Calories: 332 kcal Total Fat: 29g Total Carbs: 4.8 Protein: 12g

Pumpkin Pie Cupcakes

Preparation time: 30 minutes

Cooking time: 30 minutes

Servings: 6

Ingredients:

- 45 ml coconut flour
- 5 ml pumpkin pie spice
- 1.25 ml baking powder
- 1.25 ml baking soda
- Pinch salt
- 175 ml pumpkin puree
- 75 ml swerve brown
- 60 ml heavy whipping cream
- 1 egg
- 2.5 ml vanilla

Directions:

1. Line 6 muffin cups with parchment paper and preheat the oven to 175°C.
2. In a bowl, whisk together the salt, baking soda, baking powder, pumpkin pie spice, and coconut flour.
3. In another bowl, whisk egg, vanilla, cream, sweetener, and pumpkin puree until mixed. Whisk in dry ingredients.
4. Pour into the muffin cups and bake for about 25 to 30 minutes until it is puffed and almost set.
5. Remove and cool.
6. Refrigerate for about 1 hour.
7. Top with whipped cream and serve.

Nutrition: Calories: 70 kcal Fat: 4.1g Carb: 5.1g Protein: 1.7g

---

Brownies

Preparation time: 20 minutes

Cooking time: 20 minutes

Servings: 16

Ingredients:

- 125 ml butter, melted
- 150 ml swerve sweetener
- 3 eggs
- 2.5 ml vanilla extract
- 125 ml almond flour
- 75 ml cocoa powder
- 15 ml gelatin
- 2.5 ml baking powder
- 1.25 ml salt
- 60 ml water
- 75 ml sugar-free chocolate chips

Directions:

1. Grease an, (8 x 8-inch) baking pan and preheat the oven to 175°C.
2. In a bowl, whisk together eggs, vanilla extract, sweetener, and butter.
3. Add the salt, baking powder, gelatin, cocoa powder, and flour and whisk until combined. Stir in the chocolate chips.
4. Fill the prepared baking pan with the batter.
5. Bake for about 15 to 20 minutes until the center is still slightly wet but its edges are set.
6. Remove, cool, slice, and serve.

Nutrition: Calories: 110 kcal Fat: 9.5g Carb: 3.6g Protein: 3.1g

Ice Cream

Preparation time: 15 minutes

Cooking time: 30 minutes

Servings: 8

Ingredients:

- 575 ml heavy whipping cream, divided
- 60 ml swerve brown
- 60 ml sugar substitute
- 30 ml butter
- 12.5 ml maple extract
- 1.25 ml xanthan gum
- 75 ml chopped walnuts

Directions:

1. In a saucepan, bring two sweeteners, and 310 ml of the whipping cream to a simmer. Lower heat and gently simmer for 30 minutes.
2. Remove from the heat and whisk in maple extract and butter. Add the xanthan gum and whisk to mix well. Cool, then place in the refrigerator for about 2 hours.
3. Beat the remaining whipping cream in a bowl until stiff peaks. Foil in chilled cream/maple until well combined. Stir in chopped walnuts.
4. Freeze until firm and serve.

Nutrition: Calories: 318 kcal Fat: 31.7g Carb: 2.9g Protein: 2.8g

---

Fresh Berries with Cream

Preparation time: 10 minutes

Cooking time: 0 minutes

Servings: 4

Ingredients:

- 450 ml of coconut cream
- 45g of strawberries
- 30g of raspberries
- 15g of blueberries
- 1.25 ml of vanilla extract

Directions:

1. Put coconut cream and vanilla in the blender. Toss in the berries and blend until smooth.
2. Freeze and enjoy.

Nutrition: Calories: 303 kcal Total Fat: 28.9g Total Carbs: 12g Protein: 3.3g

---

Keto Brownies

Preparation time: 30 minutes

Cooking time: 15 minutes

Servings: 12

Ingredients:

- 170g coconut oil; melted
- 115g cream cheese
- 75 ml swerve
- 6 eggs
- 10 ml vanilla
- 85g cocoa powder
- 2.5 ml baking powder

Directions:

1. In a blender, mix eggs with coconut oil, cocoa powder, baking powder, vanilla, cream cheese, and swerve and stir using a mixer.
2. Pour this into a lined baking dish, introduce in the oven at 175° C and bake for 20 minutes
3. Slice into rectangle pieces when their cold and serve

Nutrition: Calories: 178 kcal Fat: 14g Fiber: 2g Carbs: 3g Protein: 5g

---

Keto Creamy Granola

Preparation time: 10 minutes

Cooking time: 0 minutes

Servings: 2

Ingredients:

- 225g almonds
- 75 ml coconut oil
- 75 ml sesame seeds
- 125 ml sunflower seeds
- 125 ml almond flour
- 250 ml flaxseed
- 15 ml cinnamon
- 250 ml water

Directions:

1. Preheat the oven to 148°C, and line a baking sheet with foil, then spray with baking spray. Put all nuts in a food processor to grind them slightly. Put onto the sheet, and roast in the oven for 20 minutes.
2. Take out and stir, then return and roast for another 20 minutes. Take it out and let it cool.
3. Enjoy with Greek yogurt.

Nutrition: Calories: 214 kcal Total Fat: 22g   Total Carbs: 10g Protein: 13g

Keto Popsicle

Preparation time: 20 minutes

Cooking time: 0 minutes

Servings: 2

Ingredients:

- 60 ml of heavy cream
- 30 ml of erythritol or any other Keto sweetener
- 5 ml of vanilla extract
- 250 ml of coconut milk
- 125 ml of almond milk

Directions:

1. Pour the vanilla extract and erythritol into the blender. Then add the milks and the heavy cream. Blend for 10 to 20 seconds. Get out the popsicle ice tray. Pour in the liquid, put in ice cream sticks, and freeze.
2. Enjoy when set and chilled.

Nutrition: Calories: 246 kcal Total Fat: 93g   Total Carbs: 14g Protein: 42g

---

Special Keto Pudding

Preparation time: 40 minutes

Cooking time: 5 minutes

Servings: 2

Ingredients:

- 250 ml coconut milk
- 20 ml gelatin
- 1.25 ml ground ginger
- 1.25 ml liquid stevia
- A pinch ground nutmeg
- A pinch ground cardamom

Directions:

1. In a bowl, mix 60 ml milk with gelatin and stir well.
2. Put the rest of the coconut milk in a pot and heat moderately.
3. Add gelatin mix; stir, take off heat; leave aside to cool down and then keep in the fridge for 4 hours.
4. Transfer this to a food processor, add stevia, cardamom, nutmeg and ginger then blend for some minutes Divide into dessert cups and serve cold.

Nutrition: Calories: 150 kcal Fat: 1g Fiber: 0g Carbs: 2g Protein: 6g

Keto Cheesecakes

Preparation time: 25 minutes

Cooking time: 15 minutes

Servings: 9

Ingredients:

For the cheesecakes:

- 30 ml butter
- 15 ml sugar-free caramel syrup
- 45 ml coffee
- 225g cream cheese
- 75 ml swerve
- 3 eggs

For the frosting:

- 225g soft mascarpone cheese
- 45 ml sugar-free caramel syrup
- 30 ml swerve
- 45 ml butter

Directions:

1. In your blender, mix cream cheese with eggs, 30 ml butter, coffee, 15 ml caramel syrup, and 75 ml swerve and pulse very well.
2. Spoon this into a cupcakes pan, introduce in the oven at 175° C and bake for 15 minutes
3. Leave aside to cool down and then keep in the freezer for 3 hours
4. Meanwhile; in a bowl, mix 45 ml butter with 45 ml caramel syrup, 30 ml swerve, and mascarpone cheese and blend well.
5. Spoon this over cheesecakes and serve them.

Nutrition: Calories: 254 kcal Fat: 23g Fiber: 0g Carbs: 1g Protein: 5g

Cocoa Brownies

Preparation time: 20 minutes

Cooking time: 20 minutes

Servings: 9

Ingredients:

- 125 ml salted butter, melted
- 250 ml granular swerve sweetener
- 2 large eggs
- 30 ml vanilla extract
- 12 squares melted unsweetened baking chocolate
- 10 ml coconut flour
- 30 ml cocoa powder
- 7.5 ml baking powder
- 7.5 ml salt
- 125 ml walnuts, chopped (optional)

Directions:

1. Preheat the oven to 175° C.
2. Spray the square baking pan with cooking spray or grease the pan well with butter.
3. In a large mixing bowl, use an electric mixer or whisk and mix butter and sweetener.
4. Add the eggs and vanilla extract to the bowl and mix with an electric mixer for 1 minute until smooth. Add melted chocolate and stir with a wooden spoon or spatula until the chocolate is incorporated into the butter mixture.
5. In a separate bowl, mix the dry ingredients (remaining ingredients besides walnuts) until combined.
6. Add dry ingredients into the bowl with the wet ingredients and stir with a wooden spoon until combined.
7. Add walnuts if you like.

8. Pour batter into the prepared pan. Spread to cover the entire bottom of the pan and corners.
9. Place it at the center rack of the oven and bake for 30 minutes.
10. After you've baked the brownies, take them out, and leave them in the pan to cool.
11. When cool, cut them into 9 servings, and they are ready to eat.
12. These have to be a once-in-a-while treat because they are sweet, and if you're like me, that sugar will continue to call your name. These are so good you will have to work to eat only one serving.

Nutrition: Calories: 201 kcal Carbohydrates: 5g Protein: 3g Fat: 19g

---

Raspberry and Coconut

Preparation time: 15 minutes

Cooking time: 15 minutes

Servings: 12

Ingredients:

- 60 ml of swerve
- 125 ml of coconut oil
- 125 ml of dried raspberries
- 125 ml of shredded coconut
- 125 ml of coconut butter

Directions:

1. In your food processor, blend dried berries very well.
2. Moderately heat the pan with the butter.
3. Add coconut oil, and swerve.
4. Stir and cook for 5 minutes
5. Pour half of this into a lined baking pan and spread well.
6. Add raspberry powder and also spread.
7. Top with the rest of the butter mix, spread, and keep in the fridge for a while. Cut into pieces and serve.

Nutrition: Calories: 234 kcal Fat: 22g Fiber: 2g Carbs: 4g Protein: 2g

Keto Sorbet

Preparation time: 20 minutes

Cooking time: 0 minutes

Servings: 2

Ingredients:

- 150 ml of lemon
- 250 ml of frozen blackberries
- 250 ml of frozen raspberries
- 15 ml stevia
- 250 ml water

Directions:

1. Place lemon, blackberries, raspberries, stevia and water in a blender.
2. Blend till smooth, and Keep in the freezer to harden

Nutrition: Calories: 332 kcal Total Fat: 29g Total Carbs: 4.8g Protein: 12g

---

Chocolate Chip Cookies

Preparation time: 15 minutes

Cooking time: 30 minutes

Servings: 24 cookies

Ingredients:

- 1125 ml almond flour
- 5 ml baking powder
- 2.5 ml salt
- 125 ml butter, softened
- 125 ml stevia
- 5 ml of vanilla extract
- 1 large egg
- 250 ml sugar-free chocolate chips
- 125 ml nuts, chopped

Directions:

1. Preheat the oven to 175° C.
2. Grease cookie sheets with butter and set aside.
3. In a large bowl, cream the butter and the stevia together.
4. Add the large egg and vanilla extract to the butter and stevia.
5. Mix until you incorporate the egg into the butter.
6. In a second bowl, mix almond flour, baking powder, and salt together until they mixed well.
7. Add dry ingredients to the large bowl and mix until it is combined.
8. Add sugar-free chocolate chips and nuts and stir until they are distributed evenly.
9. Drop by spoonfuls onto the cookie sheet.
10. Bake until golden brown and the surface of cookies appear dry on the top and are cooked all the way through.
11. Remove cookies from a sheet to a wire rack to cool.
12. Make these with or without nuts. We can use cocoa nibs in place of the sugar-free chocolate chips. This is a good recipe to keep on hand so

you can have a cookie along with everyone else. Make it a fun project with kids or friends. Baking is always an enjoyable way to bring people together, and this a recipe everyone will enjoy.

Nutrition: Calories: 120 kcal Carbohydrates: 3g Protein: 2g Fat: 11g
---

4-Week Meal Plan

Week 1

Week 1	Saturday	Sunday	Monday	Tuesday	Wednesday	Thursday	Friday
Breakfast	Mayonnaise Waffles	Baked Eggs	Crêpes with Lemon-Buttery Syrup	Bacon Avocado Bombs	Shrimp and Olives Pan	Baked Eggs	Mayonnaise Waffles
Lunch	Easy Mayo Salmon	Veggie, Bacon, and Egg Dish	Hot Spicy Chicken	Keto Teriyaki Chicken	Zesty Avocado and Lettuce Salad	Keto Buffalo Chicken Empanadas	Broccoli and Turkey Dish
Dinner	Mexican Shredded Beef	Creamy Chicken Bake	Balsamic Steaks	Broccoli and Chicken Casserole	Beef Stew	Simple Keto Fried Chicken	Baked Jerked Chicken
Dessert	Keto Sorbet	Chocolate Chip Cookies	Keto Creamy Granola	Keto Popsicle	Keto Popsicle	Brownies	Special Keto Pudding

Week 2

Week 2	Saturday	Sunday	Monday	Tuesday	Wednesday	Thursday	Friday
Breakfast	Coconut Macadamia Bars	Shrimp and Olives Pan	Yogurt Waffles	Baked Eggs	Bacon Avocado Bombs	Mayonnaise Waffles	Tofu & Mushroom Muffins
Lunch	Broccoli and Turkey Dish	Pepperoni and Cheddar Stromboli	Keto Teriyaki Chicken	Zesty Avocado and Lettuce Salad	Easy Mayo Salmon	Keto Buffalo Chicken Empanadas	Hot Spicy Chicken
Dinner	Chicken Schnitzel	Beef Stew	Balsamic Steaks	Broccoli and Chicken Casserole	Simple Keto Fried Chicken	Creamy Chicken Bake	Mexican Shredded Beef
Dessert	Keto Popsicle	Pumpkin Pie Cupcakes	Brownies	Raspberry and Coconut	Keto Creamy Granola	Keto Cheesecakes	Chocolate Chip Cookies

Week 3

Week 3	Saturday	Sunday	Monday	Tuesday	Wednesday	Thursday	Friday
Breakfast	Turmeric Muffins	Chicken, Bacon, Avocado Caesar Salad	Bacon Omelet	Tofu & Mushroom Muffins	Mayonnaise Waffles	Bacon Avocado Bombs	Yogurt Waffles
Lunch	Zucchini Sushi	Keto Buffalo Chicken Empanadas	California Burger Bowls	Broccoli and Turkey Dish	Zesty Avocado and Lettuce Salad	Easy Mayo Salmon	Keto Teriyaki Chicken
Dinner	Broccoli and Chicken Casserole	Baked Jerked Chicken	Sausage Stuffed Zucchini Boats	Balsamic Steaks	Simple Keto Fried Chicken	Mexican Shredded Beef	Beef Stew
Dessert	Chocolate Chip Cookies	Raspberry and Coconut	Brownies	Keto Popsicle	Cocoa Brownies	Keto Brownies	Fresh Berries with Cream

Week 4

Week 4	Saturday	Sunday	Monday	Tuesday	Wednesday	Thursday	Friday
Breakfast	Bacon Avocado Bombs	Tofu & Mushroom Muffins	Bell Pepper Frittata	Shrimp and Olives Pan	Mayonnaise Waffles	Yogurt Waffles	Bacon Avocado Bombs
Lunch	Caprese Zoodles	Zesty Avocado and Lettuce Salad	Parmesan Brussels Sprouts Salad	Keto Teriyaki Chicken	Broccoli and Turkey Dish	Keto Buffalo Chicken Empanadas	Easy Mayo Salmon
Dinner	Crispy Peanut Tofu and Cauliflower Rice Stir-Fry	Simple Keto Fried Chicken	Salmon & Shrimp Stew	Balsamic Steaks	Broccoli and Chicken Casserole	Mexican Shredded Beef	Baked Jerked Chicken
Dessert	Keto Sorbet	Brownies	Raspberry and Coconut	Ice Cream	Chocolate Chip Cookies	Cocoa Brownies	Fresh Berries with Cream

BONUS: Approved Food List for The Ketotarian

You will find many of these products throughout your new cookbook.

Olive Oil: Olive oil is versatile, delicious, and good for your health. Research shows that olive oil helps prevent cardiovascular disease by protecting your vascular system's integrity and lowering LDL - the 'bad' cholesterol. Furthermore, after new research, extra-virgin olive oil also improves the gut microbiome by increasing probiotic "Bifidobacteria" strains.

Monounsaturated fats, like olive oil, are also linked with better blood sugar regulation, including lower fasting glucose and reducing inflammation throughout the body.

Coconut Oil: The oil is also used as one of the best ways to improve ketone levels in people with nervous system disorders, such as Alzheimer's. Coconut oil contains MCTs, which speed up the ketosis process. Unlike many other fats, the MCTs are absorbed rapidly and go directly to the liver, where they are used for immediate energy – resulting in conversion to ketones.

The oil contains four types of these fats, 50% of which comes from lauric acid. Research has indicated a higher percentage may produce sustained ketosis levels because it is metabolized more gradually than other MCTs. Add coconut oil slowly to your diet because it can cause stomach cramping or diarrhea until you adjust. Begin with 5 ml daily, and work it up to 10 to 15 ml for about one week.

Meat & Poultry: Grass-fed beef (red meat) is the healthiest choice.

Eggs are at the top of the list if you want to kick away those hunger pangs at just one gram of carbs for an egg. Protect your eyes and heart and consume vital nutrients for additional health improvements.

Low-Carb Veggies: Consume vegetables and other plants that contain fiber. It is essential to look at their 'digestible' or net carbs, the total carbs minus its fiber content. Eliminate the starchy ones, including potatoes or yams, which could send the carb counts way over your daily limits. These are some examples of how to exchange your favorite foods:

- Cauliflower can be used to replace mashed potatoes or rice.
- Have a bowl of "zoodles" from zucchini with your favorite pasta.
- Spaghetti squash can replace starch store-bought spaghetti - naturally.

Put these on your shopping list of vital keto foods:

- Asparagus
- Avocado
- Broccoli
- Cabbage
- Cauliflower
- Cucumber
- Green beans
- Eggplant
- Kale
- Lettuce
- Olives
- Peppers (#1 choice is green)
- Spinach
- Tomatoes
- Zucchini

Seafood: Enjoy fish and shellfish, including salmon and others rich in Vitamin B selenium, potassium, and are almost carb-free. These are some of the grams you should be aware of before you plan the menu. For a 100-gram/ portion, you will have the following carbs:

- Oysters: 3 grams
- Clams: 4 grams
- Squid: 3 grams
- Octopus: 4 grams
- Mussels: 4 grams

If you are obese or overweight, the omega-3 fats found in Salmon, mackerel, sardines, and others are good options. According to The American Heart Association, you should consume one to two seafood meals weekly.

Cheese: You can use cheese, but you need to use caution when you make the selection. Cheese is rich in calcium, fatty acids, and protein, which are vital to your health. Consider these for your keto-friendly option:

- *Blue Cheese*: This delicious 'stinky' cheese will give you the flavor of 0.2 carbs for a small cube @ 10g It is 2 grams of protein, 2 ½ grams of fat, and 32 calories.
- *Brie*: The melting cheese is rated with 0.1 grams of carbs for 28g with 8 grams of fat and 6 grams of protein.
- *Cottage cheese*: Use caution with this one at 5-6 grams for a 125 ml portion.
- *Cream Cheese*: Use the sweet flavor provided by cream cheese at 1.6 grams of carbs for 30 ml with 10 grams of fat and 2 grams of protein. It's delicious as the main component of cheesecake and other delightful keto treats.
- *Feta*: Goat's milk is used to make feta. For each 60 ml portion, you have 1.5 grams of carbs (net) since there is no fiber. You will also get 6 grams of fat and 4 grams of protein.
- *Gruyere Cheese*: Enjoy this one with only 0.1 grams of carbs per 28g with 9 grams of fat, and 8.5 grams of protein. It's delicious on frittatas, omelets, and more.

- *Halloumi*: The grilling cheese is about one gram of carbs per 28g with 6 grams of protein and 7 grams of fat.

- *Paneer*: Indian food will incorporate paneer to its dishes with 1 gram of carbs for a 1-inch cube, which provides 7 grams of fat and 6 of protein.

- *Parmesan Cheese*: The nutty and salty flavor of parmesan equals 26 calories. It also has 1.7 grams of fat, 50 grams of protein, and 0.9 grams of carbs (per 15 ml).

- *Romano*: You can use this hard, grater-friendly cheese in your salads and other dishes as you would with parmesan. For 60 ml of shredded cheese, you should have only about 1 gram of carbs with 7 grams of fat and 9 grams of protein.

Also, Consider These Options:

- Camembert
- Cheddar
- Chevre
- Colby jack
- Havarti
- Limburger
- Manchego
- Mascarpone
- Mozzarella
- Muenster
- Pepper jack
- Provolone
- String cheese
- Swiss

Please Note: Some cheese that is forbidden include spray/canned cheese, American cheese, yellow cheddar cheese, ricotta cheese. You can have them, but they are loaded in carbs. It is best to use them in your keto recipes at a minimum.

Fresh Seeds: Increase your magnesium intake with a portion of pumpkin seeds. They help immensely with your blood sugar levels and muscles. Increase your omega-3 fatty acids with a serving of flaxseeds. The micronutrients found in flax help reduce inflammation in your body. Sesame seeds, chia seeds, or psyllium are also good options.

Fresh Nuts: Nuts are generally rich in fats with low-carb content. Nutritionists often recommend the incorporation of nuts in the keto diet. The high amount of digestible fiber in most nuts gives you a feeling of fullness upon consumption, making your body absorb a few calories in the long-run. Older women with a regular intake of nuts are known to have a low risk of mental and health diseases, as well as an excellent weight despite their old age.

Different nuts have varying levels of net carbs. Therefore, you need to know the amount of carbs present before consuming them. Nuts have more minerals than many other foods. Almonds, hazelnuts, macadamia, pecans, pine nuts, cashews, or pistachios are good choices.

Brazil nuts are very high in selenium, vital for your immune system, and help your thyroid function. Add Brazil nuts to snack time for your daily needs of selenium. Walnuts are another excellent source of omega-3 fatty acids, protein, and fiber. The combo will fill you up and prevent blood sugar spikes.

Now, Let's Move On to Cooking!

Printed in Great Britain
by Amazon